THE QUEEN'S UNIVERSITY OF BELFAST

Computers and Health

TONY GREENFIELD
Professor of Medical Statistics

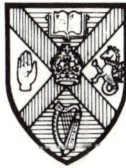

An Inaugural Lecture
delivered before the Queen's University of Belfast
on 2 December 1980

NEW LECTURE SERIES No. 125
ISBN 0 85389 190 7

Printed by
MAYNE, BOYD & SON, LTD, BELFAST

COMPUTERS AND HEALTH

Introduction

Computers have already been used for thousands of reasons in the wide world of medicine. A good review of all their uses would not be possible in less than several volumes. I shall therefore limit this talk to a personal view: a look at just a few of those applications and implications that interest me. For this is the occasion when the local community is given the chance to find out a little about the new professor and to guess at some of the things he might do during the next few years.

I shall tell you about some of the achievements in medicine with computers, some of the things which I am sure will be achieved with computers fairly soon, and some other short term possibilities. In particular I shall describe some of the activities with which I have been or expect to be involved and some of the remarkable advances that I have found here in Belfast.

I have been in Belfast for only a few weeks so that although I have already been greatly impressed by what I have found, I confidently expect to discover many more exciting developments. I hope to meet more medical users of computers during the next few months. It may be that my simple statement here of my interest in diagnosis, for example, or the integration of patient records, will prompt an introduction that will lead to mutually useful work.

Finally I shall comment on some popular anxieties that are commonly expressed about computers. Perhaps I shall allay some of these anxieties, but I shall suggest some more that you should consider.

A word about my title: *Computers and Health*. I chose it to give me plenty of scope for facts and comments and discussion. For this reason, I preferred the word 'health' to 'medicine' since it has a much wider meaning. Whereas medicine and ill-health are embraced by the subject of health there is much more to health than medicine. I shall not follow the example of the recent Reith lecturer and burden you with a long dissertation about the meaning of simple words like medicine, health, and illness but will fairly assume you know what I am talking about. Time will limit me to only a brief reference to the possible use of computers in the wider scene of health but this will be a declaration of my intent to explore these possibilities in the next few years.

A computer is a machine that processes information. It is not simply a big fast calculator as some people imagine. It can do much more than calculate.

Its heart is a central processor which is connected to a memory. And that is all, apart from some devices that are needed to enter information into the computer and then to extract the processed information from it. These are called 'input' and 'output' devices and these are what the user most sees.

Although computers range in size from boxes that might fill this lecture theatre down to silicon chips only a few millimetres square, their general structure is always the same: a central processor, a memory, and input and output.

The word 'microcomputer' has come to mean a computer about the size of a typewriter or television set that can sit on a desk. Such small machines will be seen in consulting rooms and research laboratories. Computers are suited to any tasks which are well-defined and repetitive, where mass storage of structured information is needed, and where reference to the records of selected individuals is needed very quickly from massive files of records. These abilities point at once to two areas of application in the world of medicine. The first of these is administration. Here the work is much as in any other large commercial enterprise where the computer deals with payrolls, stock control and machine scheduling. The second area of application is in medical records. For the individual patient these are created in many places, such as in a maternity hospital, in general practice, and in an X-ray clinic, and in as many different ways. Computer systems already exist in some places to bring all these records together for the benefit of the patient and of the administrative services, local and national. Although so much has been achieved in these two areas, there is still more to do. But my main interests are in those further applications where minuteness of equipment or the more advanced methods of processing information, known as 'artificial intelligence', are useful.

General Practice

Let us begin, however, with the patient whose needs may well be drowned in this fascinating ocean of technical wonders. Apart from babies and casualties, the first contact most patients have with the health services is in the consulting room of their family doctor.

Information about each patient is recorded on cards, on letters and in envelopes. No matter how good the clerical system there are limitations which are admitted by many general practitioners themselves. This is why there are already so many doctors installing their own systems using micro-computers that are very cheap: only a few hundred pounds each. I met one doctor recently who had left his practice to sell the computer system that he had developed to run it. He is doing very well. Nor has the computer industry been slow in spotting a good market.

In America the pressures are greater than here. One advertisement, which appears there in medical journals, says that for only $599 a doctor can have a computerised office enabling him to store patient data for display and updating as needed. It claims to give instant recall of vital data such as drug reactions, allergies, blood types, illness and prescription history as well as stock and laboratory control and statistical analysis.

Although it must be viewed with the usual *caveat emptor*, the advertisement seems to be offering a bargain. The forces are great and there can be no doubt that within a few years there will be a microcomputer in almost every general practice.

This is now happening so quickly that there are fears that mistakes may be made. These fears are shared by the British Medical Association which recently retained a company called Scicon to report on the situation. Scicon reported in September this year[1] that an increasing proliferation of different hardware and software systems were being implemented by general practitioners.

If this were to be continued willy-nilly, they said, a point would be reached when the opportunity to benefit from a concerted approach would be lost beyond recall. As a first step towards making a concerted approach, Scicon propose a pilot scheme to equip up to 100 general practices with micro-computers for a study lasting three years.

In their preliminary study, Scicon visited about 30 practices where microprocessors were already being used. They identified four functions as the most useful. The first of these is to create an age/sex register whereby it will be possible to identify patients who exhibit some common feature.

For example, they would be able to list all patients over 65 who need influenza immunisation, or all females under five or of child bearing age who need a german measles vaccination. The benefits to preventive medicine and health care are clear. Such a register could be extended usefully to include extra features such as diseases, drugs, occupations, social classes and geography, so that patients at risk or in need of help could be identified easily by the computer.

The second function would be to monitor and control prescriptions. The problems of prescription management are well known: patients may lose cards or suffer side-effects, the pharmacist may not be able to read the doctor's handwriting, or there may be copying errors in repeat prescriptions. If the computer were used at the time of the first prescription for a patient, it could record the medication, the dose, the frequency and the dates of repeat prescriptions. It would automatically type prescriptions and thereby reduce copying and dispensing errors. It would plan and monitor recall visits so that the doctor would be able to assess clinical effects and the behaviour of the patient. It would also provide a reference system for drug interactions, costs, and side effects.

The third function would be to record, retrieve, summarise and present information in a legible form whenever the patient was seeing the doctor. Thus the doctor would have before him, automatically and instantaneously, the patient's clinical and social characteristics, his medical history, drug treatments and effects.

The fourth function is that which many doctors may be tempted to put first on their list. It is to use computers to do the practice housekeeping. It can control appointments, for example, compute fees, salaries and wages, and control stocks of drugs and other consumables. It can be used to analyse prescribing patterns or the workload of partners, to evaluate trainee schemes and to maintain the patient lists of health visitors. It can be used for word processing: writing standard letters, reports, forms and lists. It could print labels: for letters to patients or to put on samples sent away for testing. Labels on samples could be in a form that would enable another machine to read them so as to reduce the chances of laboratory mixups.

A more remote but potentially valuable use of computers in general practice that Scicon identified was to communicate with other systems. For example, it may be used to obtain information from the National Formulary or from libraries of clinical research reports. It may be used to transfer information about individual patients from and into hospital records and so accelerate the service to those patients. Or the doctor may be able to refer to patient records while out on his rounds, using a portable terminal and an ordinary telephone line.

Overall, the advantages to the doctor are: savings in administrative and clerical effort and costs, and more efficient and effective management of the practice. The advantages to the patient are: early warnings of risks, recall notices, better prescription control, and better care resulting from analysis of information.

While there can be little argument about the benefits of these small computers to general practice, Scicon advise: "Make haste slowly". For it is clear that a concerted and standardised approach is essential and until many possibilities have been examined and tested, that standard approach cannot be specified.

However, to those general practitioners who cannot wait for these wonders my advice is: read the Scicon report to the BMA because it contains sound practical technical advice that will help you greatly.

What are the deterrents? Cost cannot be one of them since small systems to provide age/sex and contacts registers can be had, fully programmed, for less than £1,000. Larger systems for group practices, to fulfil many of the functions I have described, including recall facilities for such needs as cervical smears, tetanus, polio and german measles immunisation, hypertension and diabetes, may cost up to £20,000, but no more.

Another deterrent is the expected need for training. Most doctors have no wish to learn how to program a computer. But nor do they need to, for the computers will come already programmed and with simple working instructions. Certainly an appreciation of computer capabilities would be valuable to anyone who intends to use a computer. It is already a requirement of the medical statistics department of Queen's University to teach all medical undergraduates some little appreciation of the use of computers.

But the new generation of doctors will need a more thorough understanding of computers, of how they work, how to use them, and of their many applications. I hope that my department will contribute to meeting this need.

One application of computers in general practice that I have not mentioned so far is in diagnosis of illness. This, you might argue, should be the first use to be considered because it is certainly the problem that dominates the minds of most patients when they ask: "Doctor, what is wrong with me?" It is also a problem that doctors readily acknowledge since there are so many conditions that cannot be diagnosed without doing tests and without specialised knowledge. That is why doctors refer patients to hospitals. But computers can and do already help with diagnosis. I shall describe some of the ways in which they do this later in this lecture. But computer diagnosis is at present limited mainly to special conditions and it will be a few years before general diagnosis systems will be available. However, before the end of the century I am sure that most family doctors will be using small computers to help them with diagnosis, in deciding what further tests need to be done, and in prescribing treatment. The real cost here is not in the equipment but in the research that must be done to formulate the decision rules for the computer to use. Perhaps the drug companies, as well as the small computer makers, will lead the investment here because they have so much to gain from the close relationship between diagnosis and pre-scription. The benefits to the patient of earlier and more accurate diagnosis are clear.

Hospitals

The amount of information in an urban hospital is beyond human imagination. There are records not only for the hundreds of in-patients but also for the tens of thousands of out-patients over many years. The storage and processing of all this information is formidable, yet to a degree it works because good administrative and clerical systems have been developed. But this was the first area to which computers were applied in some health services. Over the last 25 years work has proceeded in automating record systems for separate departments lead-ing in some hospitals to total information systems.

Administrative needs have usually been put first, perhaps because the administrators control the finances. This may not seem to be putting the patient's needs high, but administration has become the basis for total information systems. In the long run this is good for the patients as is seen by the sequence of development in some American hospitals. Money is openly acknowledged to be important in America so the early computer systems designed there were aimed at tracking a patient as he progressed through the many parts of the hospital. This made it possible to build an item-by-item account to be presented to him, or his widow, later. This may be one of the reasons why the Americans seem to be ahead in using computers in hospital information systems.

For once a patient tracking and costing system has been created it is not such a big step to give piggybacks to clinically useful information. Thus a system that is first created for the benefit of administration, for financial and technical management, can be extended to collect and supply information from and to say, biochemical analysis laboratories, intensive care units, or interactive terminals used by consultants, or ward nurses.

More generally, however, applications of computers have been developed by separate departments, working independently of each other so that while each may have made good progress the problem of integrating their work has arisen. This is a problem to which the hospitals of Northern Ireland should give their attention and I hope that my department may be of service. Nevertheless, all these developments have been made with benefits to the patients in view to help with his diagnosis, his treatment, and in following his progress and I shall describe some of them.

Biochemistry

There are few people who have never had a blood test. It has become almost routine for a doctor to arrange for a patient to give a sample of his blood to be analysed. Not many years ago, chemists analysed blood by hand. But as the diagnostic value of blood analysis increased, so did the demands by doctors, so that the analytical chemist had to apply the factory techniques of mass production. In the Royal Victoria Hospital, for example, the biochemistry department does about 15,000 analyses every day from 750 samples of blood. This is possible only by using automatic analysis which is controlled by computer.

The automatic equipment is known as SMAC, which stands for Sequential Multiple Analyser with Computer. In the analytical console of SMAC the specimens are taken up a central riser, from which drops flow through 12 analytical channels on each side: 24 in all. Each of these channels is equipped to sense the concentration of a specific component of blood serum by a colour measuring technique. Four of the channels are used for control so that SMAC measures 20 components of serum. The signals are sent to the computer which has a screen, on which the analysis can be shown, and a printer. The signals are sent on to the laboratory's central computer which produces a report to be returned to the doctor for his interpretation. This equipment has brought great advantages to biochemical analysis. Speed, accuracy and precision are three, but stamina is another. For no human being could reasonably be expected to maintain such a rate of analysis, with such boring repetition, for so long, without at least complaining, and probably making mistakes.

So that is another advantage of a computer controlled method: it makes very few mistakes.

Further development is clearly to link the output of this small computer to a central medical information system so that results are transmitted instantaneously to the point where they can be used. Also so that the results can be stored immediately for recall and use later. A further advantage of direct linking with the central computer is that it is there that the data can be used to help with diagnosis.

Since the work some statisticians have contributed to improving diagnosis is so closely related to blood analysis, I shall describe one of the several methods here.

But common to all methods is the general idea of giving the computer information about lots of well people and lots of ill people and teaching it how to tell one from the other. Then when the individual patient is examined, the computer is able to decide which type of person he is: if he is ill or well, and if he is ill in what way.

The standard practice with analytical results is to refer to normal ranges. For example, if your serum calcium concentration is between 9.0 and 10.3 milligrams per 100 millilitres you would be judged to be normal, or well, so far as calcium is a guide. If your serum calcium were less than 9.0 or greater than 10.3 milligrams per 100 millilitres, you would be judged to be not normal, or unwell. The same applies to magnesium whose normal range is given by Eastham's Biochemical Values to be between 1.8 and 2.4 mg per 100 ml, and for any other component of blood serum whose normal ranges are published.

You will appreciate that the limits of these normal ranges are just practical cut-off points and that the *true* distribution of calcium concentration in normal people is more like figure one, with a small proportion of perfectly well people being a bit over the top or a bit under the bottom. However, if your doctor has asked for an analysis of calcium to confirm his tentative diagnosis that your parathyroid gland is overactive, he needs a rule to guide him.

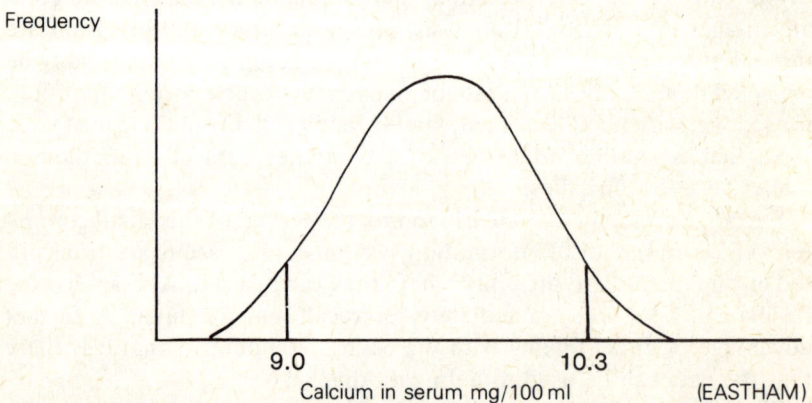

Fig. 1   The distribution of calcium concentration in the blood serum of normal people. Normal ranges given by Eastham's Biochemical Values.

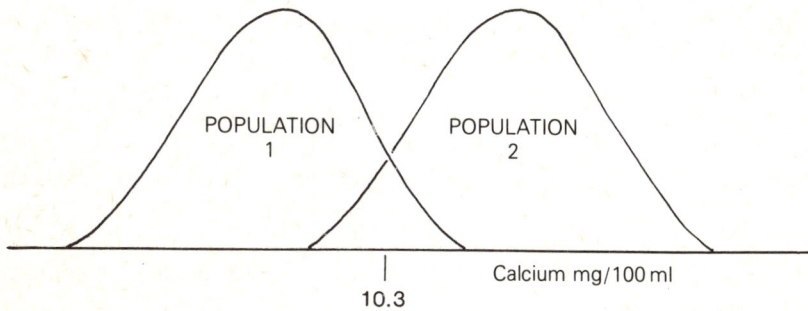

discriminant (diagnostic) rule:

if   x < 10.3 assign to population 1
if   x ≥ 10.3 assign to population 2

Fig. 2   The hypothetical distribution of serum calcium for people with over-active parathyroid glands is shown on the right.

Figure two shows the problem: if the serum calcium of people with over active parathyroid glands has the distribution on the right, and the serum calcium of normal people has the distribution on the left, then no matter where you put the cut-off point there is some chance that the diagnosis will be wrong. The statistical word for a diagnostic rule of this nature is a 'discriminant'.

The problem is increased when other components of blood are considered because, looking at them one at a time, the doctor may reach a different decision for each. It is a sad limitation of human minds that there are very few that can repeatedly and constantly judge more than one variable at a time. This is where the computer can help.

You may recall from your knowledge of the royal families of Europe that haemophilia, the bleeding disease, is experienced almost always by males and not by females, but that it is passed to the boys by their mothers who are called carriers. The diagnostic problem is to detect carriers among women so that they can be warned of the possible consequences of having male children. Here is how I tackled the problem using measurements made by the haematology department in Sheffield.

In the blood there is a substance called clotting factor VIII-C and figure three shows the values for two sets of people. The lower line shows values for some women who are known to be carriers and the upper shows values for some women who are known to be normal. Now you can see that although the averages of the two sets of values may be different, there is a lot of overlap. The fact that a statistical test will show that the averages are different is no consolation whatever to the poor woman who wants to know whether or not she is a carrier of haemophilia and her value of factor VIII-C is somewhere in the middle of the total spread.

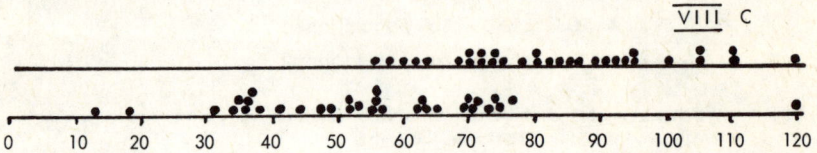

Fig. 3   Dot diagrams for clotting factor VIII-C values for two sets of people: haemophilia carriers and normals.

There is another substance in the blood called clotting factor VIII-RA and figure four shows the values for the same two sets of people. Here again there is a lot of overlap, but there is very much more than with factor VIII-C. Indeed there is so much overlap that you might reasonably argue that there could be no value whatever in considering this extra measurement. However, if we plot the two values together on a single graph, factor VIII-RA against factor VIII-C, a new picture emerges, as in figure five.

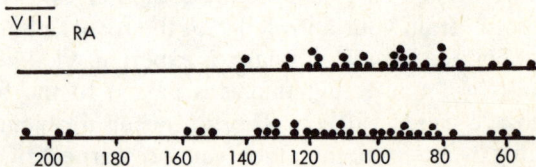

Fig. 4   Dot diagrams for clotting factor VIII-RA values for two sets of people: haemophilia carriers and normals.

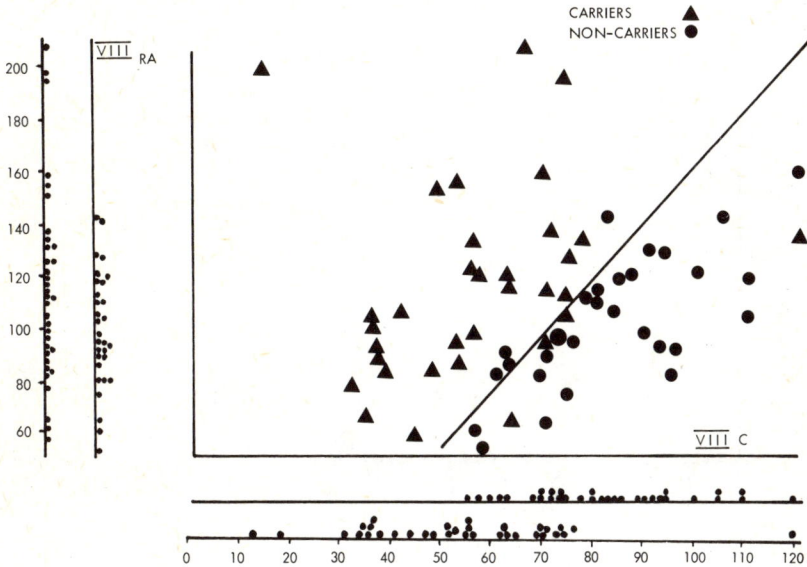

Fig. 5 A bivariate plot of the values shown in figures three and four, with a discriminant line almost completely separating the two sets of values.

Now the overlap has almost disappeared. I have preserved the original diagrams in the bottom and left margins to remind you of the confusion created by using only one variable at a time. By using both variables together it is possible to draw a line, called a discriminant line, between the two sets of points.

There is now so little overlap that there are very few points on the wrong sides of the discriminant line. We are fortunate in this case that a good diagnostic rule can be found using only two variables so that it can be represented as a diagnostic chart as in figure six.

The diagnostic chart is used by the consultant to guide him in making a diagnosis of an individual using two measured quantities. As well as pointing to the most likely diagnosis, the chart also tells the doctor the probability that this diagnosis is correct. It so happens that this analysis could be done by simple manual plotting because only two variables were being considered. When more than two variables are needed it is not so easy, but a computer can be used.

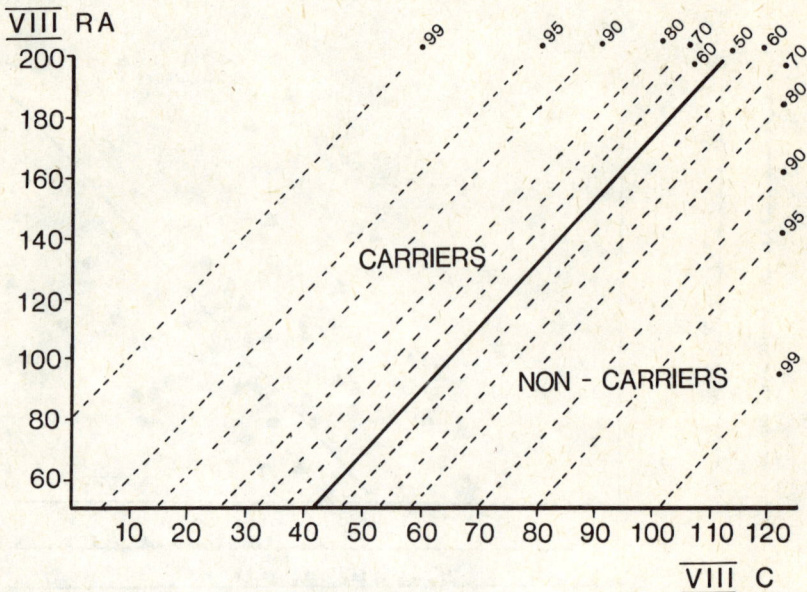

Fig. 6   A diagnostic chart for haemophiliac carriers.

One of the great anxieties about computers is that they may make mistakes. This anxiety was expressed strongly by a paediatrician who recently wrote to the British Medical Journal that he had been appalled to discover that a computer had apparently analysed a urine sample from one of his patients and then recommended a certain drug for a urinary infection. He believed the drug was the wrong one in that case because the computer had not taken into account the patient's clinical condition, nor how the urine sample was collected, and there was no conclusive proof that there was a urinary infection. Although child specialists would not act on the advice on this machine, he added, he feared that a family doctor with no specialist knowledge might give the drug without question. This could have led to side effects and the possibility of other, more appropriate drugs eventually being less successful in treating the child.

The answer usually given to this anxiety is that the system should be designed to allow a human expert to over-rule the computer. But this answer raises another anxiety: What if the computer is right and the human is wrong? Here is an example that shows that when dealing with several variables at a time, the computer is much more likely to be right than the human. This is because the human is not very good at thinking about more than one variable at a time.

There are many tests that are available to investigate the function of your thyroid gland[2].

Simply stated, there are three alternative conditions of the thyroid gland: it can be over-active, or hyperthyroid; it can be normal; or it can be under active, or hypothyroid. Several tests are available to help to diagnose your particular condition. One of these is to measure the protein-bound iodine in your blood serum in micrograms per hundred millilitres. Figure seven shows values measured for three sets of people and you can see that there is a lot of overlap between the normal and each of the other two states although there is no overlap between the hyper and the hypo. The conventional normal range is shown on this diagram by the two parallel vertical lines.

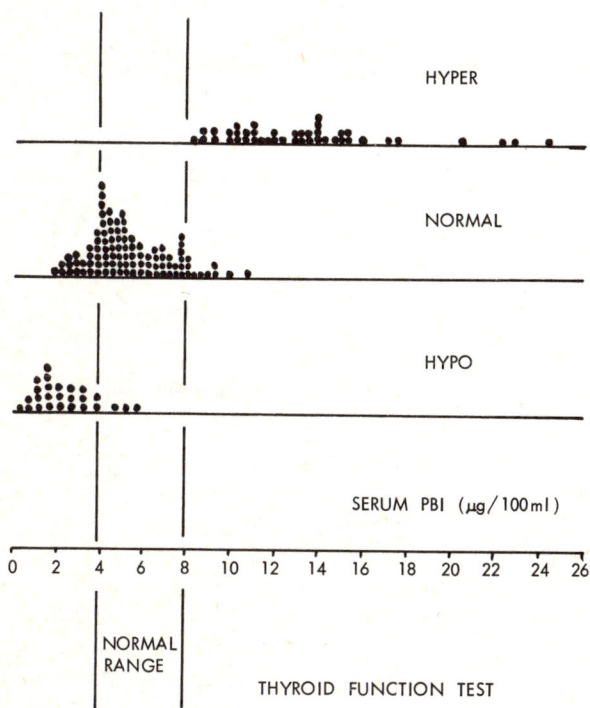

Fig. 7 Dot diagrams for protein-bound iodine for three sets of people: hyperthyroid, normal and hypothyroid.

16

Another test is to measure the percentage uptake of T-3, a hormone produced by the thyroid using a commercial product called Triosorb which was designed for this test. Figure eight shows that there is far more overlap, indeed so much that the hyper and hypo values overlap

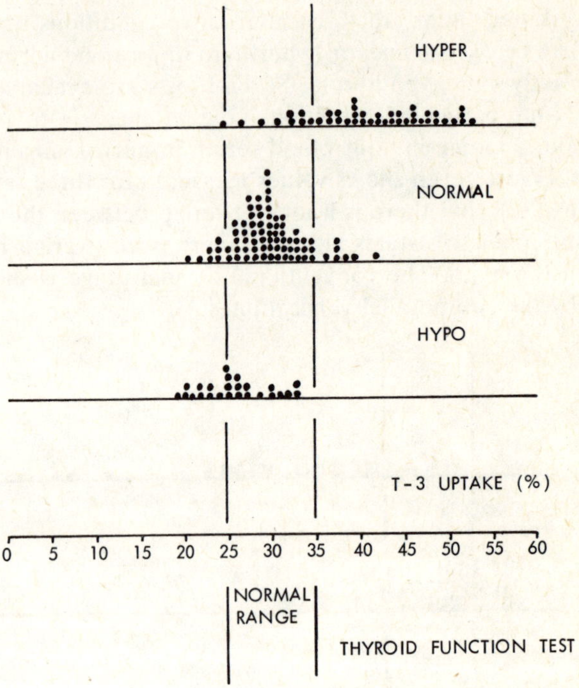

Fig. 8 Dot diagrams for T-3 uptake for three sets of people: hyperthyroid, normal, and hypothyroid.

and run into each other's territories beyond the normal ranges which are again shown by two vertical lines. How could this apparently fuzzy information possibly help to improve the chance of a good diagnosis? My answer again was to use both values together, as in figure nine.

In this diagram, the two slanting lines are the discriminants which separate the three conditions to be diagnosed. It is clear that these are far more likely to diagnose the individual patient correctly than either of the two variables treated on its own. The lines showing the normal ranges point to how their use can lead to incorrect diagnoses. Further than that, this chart has also been used to diagnose some individuals

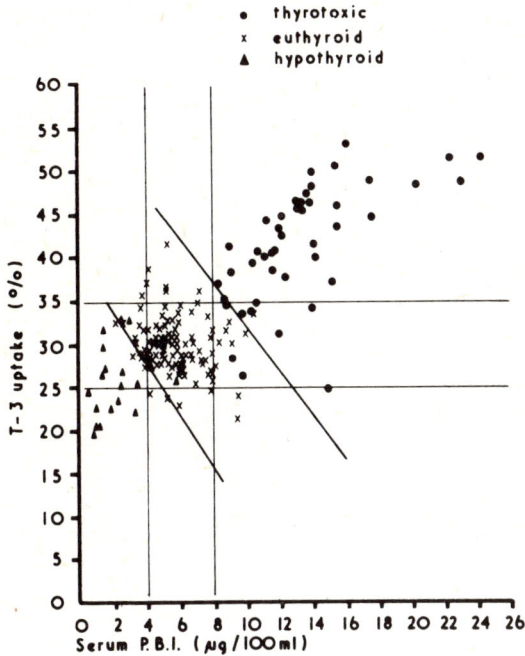

Fig. 9 A bivariate plot of the values shown in figures seven and eight, with discriminant lines separating the three sets of people.

correctly months after they had been diagnosed incorrectly. It emphasises my anxiety that the human being, who thinks that he is right and the machine is wrong, may over-rule the computer when in fact the computer is right.

In both these cases I have been able to use pictures to illustrate the value of the computer in diagnosis because in each case two variables were enough. However, most diagnostic situations need more, sometimes many more, than two variables and here there is no question that the computer can perform better than the human in considering all the variables together so long as the right variables are being used. This is the practical answer to the paediatrician's concern about misdiagnosis by the computer of a urinary infection: we must ensure that enough of the right information is available.

The ability of the computer to cope with many variables at once is also useful when it is asked to analyse images. It can, for example, look at the radio-isotope image of a brain and, ignoring all the normal features, tell us when an abnormal feature is present.

If we consider the side view of a brain in figure ten in just two parts, the front and the back, and call the average radio-isotope image-intensity for each part X_1 and X_2 respectively, these two measurements can be plotted on a graph as a single point. If we made similar measurements on 30 normal brains, we could plot all thirty pairs of values as thirty points, as in figure 11.

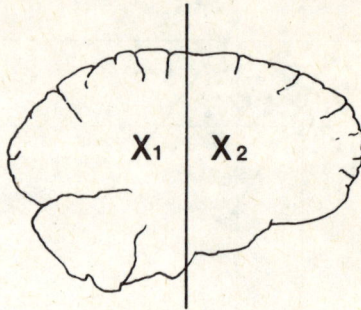

Fig. 10   A side view of a brain divided into two areas.

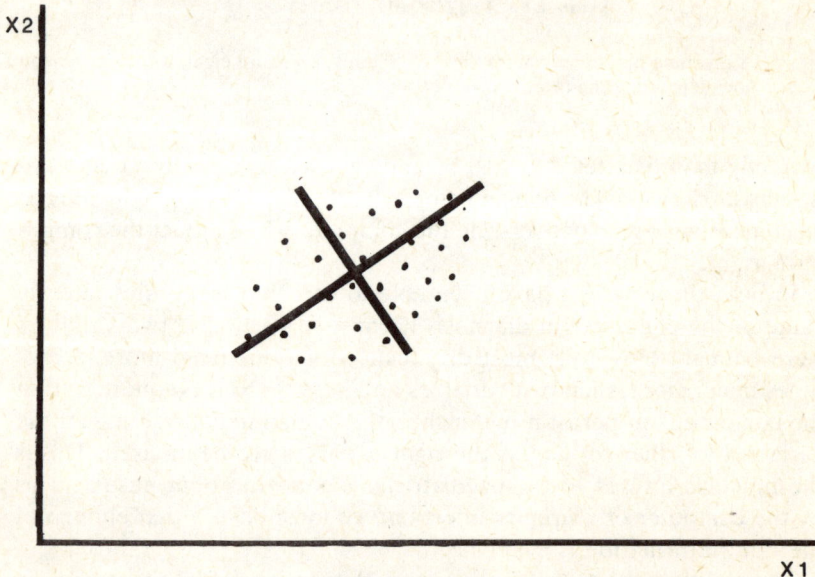

Fig. 11   A plot of radio-isotope in age intensities (X1 and X2) for 30 normal brains.

There is a statistical technique, called principal components analysis, which is used to describe an array of points. This is illustrated by the two solid lines drawn over our array of 30 points.

The longer of the two lines is in the direction of the greater variation. The shorter one is in the direction of the lesser variation. These are called the principal directions of variation between the points.

But the division of the brain into two parts only would not give us enough resolution to be able to separate any normal features from abnormal features, so consider dividing the brain into three parts instead, to give slightly better resoultion.

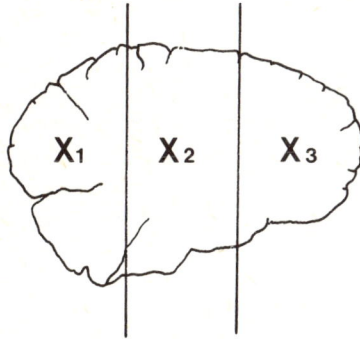

Fig. 12   A side view of a brain divided into three parts.

We can now call the average of the radio-isotope image intensity for each part X_1, X_2 and X_3 respectively so that these three measurements can be plotted in a three-dimensional graph as a single point. If enough points were plotted it would be possible to draw three lines to represent the three principal directions of variation between the points. In general, as many directions of variation may be found as there are dimensions in the data. These can be used to describe the structure of the data.

However, the division of the brain into only three areas would still give too poor a resolution to detect if anything is wrong: if the measurements from the individual brain deviate abnormally from the data structure we have for a set of normal brains.

Much greater precision is obtained by dividing the brain scan image into 60 small squares. The 60 measurements from this scan may therefore be plotted as a single point in a 60 dimensional space. Unfortunately, we humans are not able to visualise a 60-dimensional space but we are able to train a computer to do so.

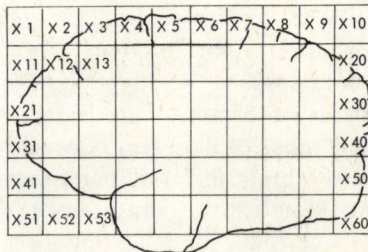

X 1	X 2	X 3	X 4	X 5	X 6	X 7	X 8	X 9	X 10
X 11	X 12	X 13							X 20
X 21									X 30
X 31									X 40
X 41									X 50
X 51	X 52	X 53							X 60

Fig. 13   A side view of a brain divided into 60 parts.

Dr David Barber[3] at Sheffield has been working with even higher resolution by producing 384 measurements from a single brain scan, so that these may be thought of as a single point in 384-dimensional space. Then, using measurements from a large number of normal brains, he used the computer to find the first 20 principal components. These were enough to describe the structure of the variation between normal individuals. When an individual patient is examined to look for some abnormality in his brain, the first twenty principal components representing normal features are subtracted from his measurements. If the remaining image is not uniformly gray, it is then easy to detect an abnormality.

Patients in the Royal Victoria Hospital of Belfast have the benefit of a miracle of the nineteen-seventies, which was the invention of computerised tomography. This is the most impressive development of all image processing systems since the discovery of X-rays. It is a technique which begins with taking several X-ray pictures of a thin slice of the human body. Each of these pictures is taken from a different angle by rotating the equipment round the patient. At each angle, the equipment moves across the body so that the section is scanned by X-rays and the image of the scan is recorded and sent into the computer. The patient is able to lie relaxed and comfortable while everything else is moving around her. When the scans are fed into the computer, it analyses them and assembles a new picture which looks as if it were taken as a full view of the section.

Figure 14 is a picture which the computer has created by putting together the X-ray scans across the patient's head at a level just above the bridge of the nose.

It is clear that cross-sectional scans like these will reveal much more diagnostic information than conventional X-rays, because they can differentiate between soft tissues and can reveal features that would normally be obscured by bone. Because the picture is digital and was created by a computer, it can be stored in the computer and can be analysed even further, using techniques of pattern recognition, to reveal

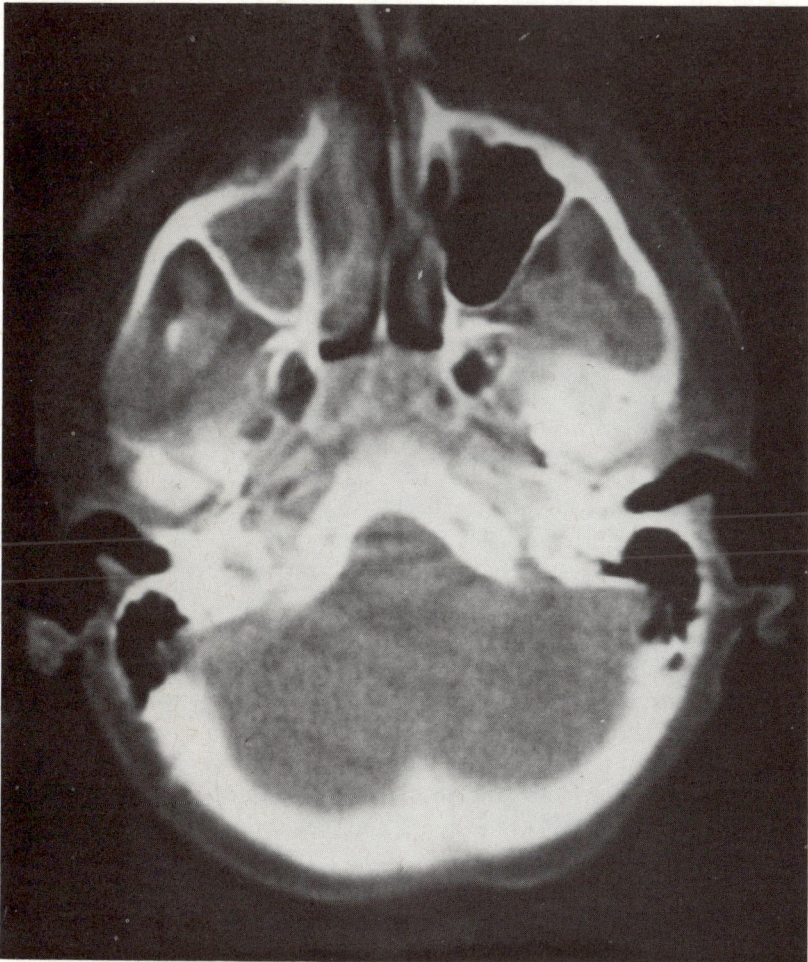

Fig. 14   A sectional view, produced by the computer, of the patient's head.

diseased areas. Mr Alan Webb, in the medical physics department at the
Royal Victoria Hospital, has made his own contribution to this work by
introducing colour to mark differences in tissue.

A slide was shown in which colour had been used with great effect to
reveal, in a section across the front half of the brain, the presence of a
meningioma, which is a cancer spreading from the membrane surrounding the brain. Not only does the coloured scan reveal the presence of the
cancer, but it also makes possible the measurement of its boundaries and
volume and its fine details, so that inferences can be made about its
nature.

Also in the Royal Victoria Hospital in Belfast, a computer is used
many times every day to help with diagnosis by recording and analysing
another kind of image which is viewed by a gamma-ray camera.

A black and white image of a pair of lungs as seen by a gamma-ray
camera is made by injecting a mildly radioactive material into a vein so
that the blood carries it through the lungs and taking a photograph to
record the intensity of radioactivity. The image can be converted into an
array of numbers, according to the intensity, and stored in a computer.
When the picture is displayed by the computer, various colours can be
used for different intensities. This immediately makes it much easier to
see that there has been a relatively poor flow of blood into the right
lung.

However, the picture can be improved even further by the computer.
As it is, the picture is rather fuzzy because of the random variation in the
radio-activity. The computer deals with this by smoothing the image and
getting rid of the fuzziness.

The smoothing process has produced a much higher quality picture.
An even cleverer use of the computer is that it can measure changes in
the way an organ is behaving over a short period of time.

For example, the computer can record a sequence of pictures to show
what happens when some radioactive material is injected into a vein in
the patient's right arm. The pictures are recorded at one second intervals
to show the material moving up the right arm, into the right half of the
heart, through the heart and into the lungs, through the lungs, and
returning to the left side of the heart, and then through the aorta into the
rest of the body.

If there were a defect in the wall that separates the two sides of the
heart, some of the blood on the left side would leak through to the right
and would be returned to the lungs too early.

To see if this is happening, the radiologist can mark a small area on the picture. He then asks the computer to plot a graph of the image intensity of that small area as it varies with time and to analyse the graph into two components. The computer tells us that the original curve is a combination of a normal lung circulation curve and a smaller premature recirculation curve. This supports the suggestion that there is a leak from the left to the right side of the heart.

Computer Interviewing

A completely different development for helping with diagnosis is in the training of computers to interview patients about their medical histories and present syptoms. Many people, when they hear of this, are horrified. Some say that it can't be done. Others say that even if it could be done, it shouldn't be done. There seems to be a widespread belief that the use of computers to interview patients will dehumanise medicine, that even if doctors accepted the use of computers, patients would never allow themselves to be interviewed by machines.

There are several answers to these objections, and they all spring from plenty of experience with well-managed trials.[4]

Some years ago the Department of Health asked the National Physical Laboratory to develop computer programs for interviewing patients and to try them out in a variety of clinical situations.

Since then there have been many trials involving over 20 hospitals or clinics in the UK and thousands of patients. These have produced several successful interview programs which have proved to be highly acceptable to both patients and doctors. It has been found that patients actually enjoy computer interviewing and recognise its value in improving communication with the doctor. The programs have been written to have a pleasing personality and avoid the social or intellectual barriers that patients sometines see in front of a doctor. There is no feeling of embarrassment either, as has been shown with a program dealing with psycho-sexual problems. Furthermore, in answering questions about their alcohol problems, patients have been more truthful and accurate than they are when questioned by a psychiatrist. From the doctor's viewpoint, the system, is seen to save a lot of time because the programs produce printed summaries of interviews which are available immediately afterwards for the doctor. These summaries are also stored for later reference and to provide a data base for later analysis to create better diagnostic rules. All of the programs developed so far have been for history taking into account conditions such as abdominal pain, back ache, ante-natal risks, breathing difficulties and industrial health.

One large private health organisation, BUPA, is using computer terminals for interviewing their clients in general health screening. There is a good story told by the medical director, Dr Alan Bailey. He introduced a woman client to a terminal and showed her how to use it. Incidentally this is very easy because there are only four buttons to touch. These are marked 'YES', 'NO', 'DON'T KNOW', and 'DON'T UNDERSTAND'. Twenty minutes after leaving her alone with the terminal he returned to find her in tears. "Oh my dear", he said, "what is the trouble?" "It's nothing at all doctor", she replied. "I'm crying because I'm so happy. I've been coming here for 15 years and this is the first time anybody has taken any notice of me". With such approval from the patients, we can be sure that this system which improves medical information, and hence medical care, must eventually win the enthusiasm of doctors who are devoted to medical care.

The computer's varied contributions to diagnosis that I have described, together with others which you may find in the literature, must be brought together into integrated systems to cover the majority of diagnostic situations. The computers that are already used to handle the mass production of blood analysis, the storing of notes taken by the doctor and by the computer, X-ray and gamma-ray cameras, the body scan machines, population statistics of diseases, and so on, should link into a central computer that will make the best use of all the pooled information.

For the aims of medicine are simple enough. They are to examine the patient and to determine if he needs some form of treatment. The treatments may be surgical, drugs, physiotherapy, radiation, nursing, exercise, diet or nothing at all. The decisions to be made are based on diagnosis, past history of the patient, his present condition other than his illness, what is known of the past history of the human race, and what treatments are available. The computer serves as a decision advising machine. As well as advising the doctor of the most probable diagnosis, it refers to stored medical history so that it can suggest the most relevant treatments. This is called a computer-based patient management system. Several such systems are already advanced in design and giving some service to hospitals. Most of them are in America, where perhaps the most advanced is MARIS[5], developed in Georgia, which uses information based on practical situations embedded in normal medical records.

The benefits to the patient are clearly an improvement in all aspects of service. The economic advantage is that if money can be saved by improving communications then more will be available to meet other needs.

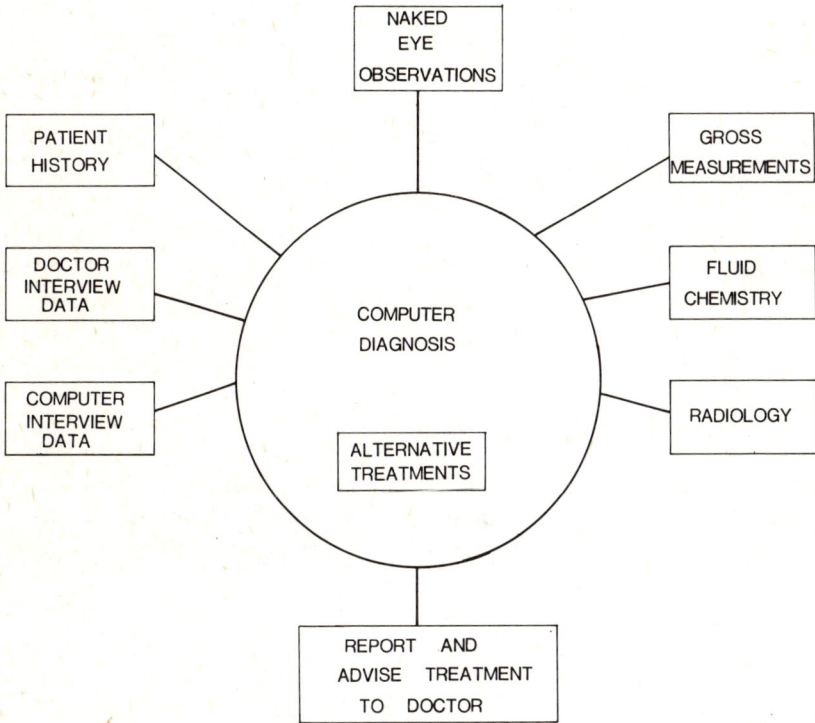

Fig. 15   A plan for the future.

A prospect that may not please the medical profession so much is that miniature mimics of these medical systems will soon be marketed for home use. There are many small computers in homes already, that have cost less than a thousand pounds each, and some that have cost less than a hundred pounds. They are being bought at present for such simple pleasures as playing games, doing household accounts, storing recipes and preparing menus. However, most people are interested in their own health and sickness and for more than a century most homes have had reference books on medicines and sickness as well as healthier pursuits of exercise and good diets.

Have no doubt that computer diagnosis in the home, together with advice for self-treatment, is on the way. It will be useless for doctors, who may see dangers in the prospect, to complain for they will be powerless to stop it because every man and woman who is so quick to self-administer thermometer, aspirin and lemon-drink will soon discover the ego-centric pleasure of communing with the home computer.

It has already started with programs to compute horoscopes and biorhythms which, to the common man, are the first steps in medication administered by the home computer. The automatic Dr Spock and other domestic hypochondriac machines are just round the corner. If you think it should be stopped but accept that it cannot be stopped, your next best course of action is to join in with the exploitation of home computer medicine and ensure that it is done in the best possible way. Let us be positive and look for the advantages. One of these may be that the computer could advise the user that his illness really is too trivial to bother the doctor about. Alternatively it may advise him that what he thinks is trivial really merits medical attention. Further benefits of home computers, or their natural extension: home or kiosk contained terminals connected to big public computers like Prestel, is that they may be useful in therapy. For example, they may be used to substitute the samaritan service. An advantage of the friendly computer is that although it is endowed with personality, it is nevertheless known by the person in trouble to be not a person and hence can be consulted more freely. This occurred to me recently when watching a television program about the increase in suicides by drug overdoses among teenagers whose complaint was that they could not talk easily to established authorities about their problems. A computerised aunt Mary may be the answer. Another advantage that is already well at work is the companionship of a small computer. There are many disabled people, blind, deaf, and paraplegic who are benefiting from an enormous number of inventions based on small computers. Many of these are for communication, to help the blind to read books or the paralysed to type messages or the deaf to use telephones.

But to some disabled people, the simple home computer itself, without being used for special applications has brought great happiness and purpose to life, bringing with it intellectual and creative occupation as well as amusing pastimes.

Much more could be said about the therapeutic prospects of small computers but for my final illustration I shall briefly describe an invention that has been made by Dr Kenneth McMullen in Queen's University of Belfast. This is a device that will automatically determine the body's need for insulin and will then deliver it to the body. The device includes a sensor to measure tissue sugar level, a pump to deliver insulin, a computer to calculate the amount of insulin needed and to control the pump, a well of concentrated insulin, and a power supply. Yet, with all these components, it will still be small enough to implant inside the body.

The computer will eventually be made to exist on one small integrated circuit so that the total device can be encapsulated for implanting. Small pumps have been designed before for delivering insulin, but not so small as this and there has been none which would automatically deliver insulin in response to direct sensing of sugar levels in tissue. Some technical problems remain before this project is completed, but the major problem is financial. We must hope that money will be found soon to enable this project to be completed because it offers such great relief to diabetic people who are about one percent of the population. For the United Kingdom alone, that means there are about half a million diabetics.

Further developments must be in similar devices that can be implanted to deliver hormones and other drugs to those in need. This is an area of invention in which I expect the major pharmaceutical companies to invest. Indeed I should not be surprised to learn that they were already well on the way.

Even if these devices are not implanted, because the cost of surgery will be a constraint, it is not far-fetched to imagine a device that will be worn like a wrist-watch that will sense your pulse, blood pressure, temperature, skin moisture, tissue oxygen and acidity. It may also measure the variables of the atmosphere surrounding you, such as the temperature, humidity, pressure, noxious gases and degree of ionisation. The watch face would not only tell you the values of all these variables but it would also compute warnings to slow down, or breathe deeply or take some exercise or have a drink and it would actuate controllers to inject a drug.

Such gadgets, as well as home computers, will be called personal health machines and I have little doubt that they will be on the market in about five years. Will they be dangerous toys? Will they impose an added load on our medical services? Or will they help to eliminate, through prevention, the need to go to the doctor or to the hospital, by preventing sickness and assuring the wearers of good health?

The flow of progress cannot be stopped. With few exceptions, the medical world recognises this and is actively encouraging and participating in the progress. There is no doubt that the health care services of the western world already rely greatly on the collection, storage, processing, and reporting of information by computers. Within a few decades, I predict, they will do so almost totally.

This has been a brief survey of what is happening in the application of computers in the health services and what is likely to happen in the near future. But I have tried to show those areas to which I hope my department will contribute during the next few years. The first of these is in teaching: to increase the appreciation among doctors of what computers can do for them. The second is in diagnosis: to bring together various special developments into a more general tool for helping clinicians. This includes the use of a computer to interview patients. The third area, to which I hope my department will contribute, is in creating a central computerised medical information system for the Belfast and Northern Ireland hospitals, linking together the many successful but unfortunately separate departmental computers that already exist.

If we can contribute in these areas I feel we shall have played a useful role in supporting the health of the people of Northern Ireland.

But one effect of computers to which all people concerned with human health should give their most serious attention is the new industrial revolution. Here I repeat a warning that was made as long ago as 1947 when the first digital computer had only recently been assembled. The warning was made by the father of cybernetics, Norbert Wiener, one of the most perceptive geniuses of the century.

"The first industrial revolution", he wrote, "the revolution of the dark satanic mills, was the devaluation of the human arm by the competition of machinery. There is no rate of pay at which a pick and shovel labourer can live which is low enough to compete with the work of a steam shovel as an excavator.

"The modern industrial revolution is similarly bound to devalue the human brain. Taking the second revolution as accomplished, the average human being of mediocre attainments or less has nothing to sell that is worth anyone's money to buy."

Wiener had realised, as the world stood in the shadow of Nagasaki and the atomic bomb, that in automation "we were in the presence of another social potentiality of unheard of importance for good and evil".

His answer was to start planning a society then, in 1947, and with urgency, that would be based on human values other than buying or selling or material production. For he knew, as we know, that we cannot stop progress. We do not want to stop progress because it has so much to offer. But we must control its worst effects. One way to do this is to concentrate our efforts on those aspects of technical progress that are for the common good.

The application of computers to medicine and health in general is an opportunity that should not be lost. It is good that the Queen's University of Belfast, together with the health services of Northern Ireland, is facing this challenge.

Acknowledgements

I thank Mr Brendan Ellis and Miss Cathy Gilmartin of the photographic unit at the Royal Victoria Hospital for their excellent artwork and slides.

I also thank Mr Desmond Neill of the Biochemistry department, Dr Rodney Ferguson and Mr Alan Webb of the Medical Physics department at the Royal Victoria Hospital, and Dr Kenneth McMullen of the Belfast City Hospital, for their kind help in preparing this lecture and for providing some slides.

References

(1) Palmer, P., Rees, C.: *Computing in General Practice* (Prepared by Scicon for the General Medical Services Committee of The British Medical Association, September 1980).
(2) Barnett, D. B. *et al: Discriminant Value of Thyroid Function Tests.* British Medical Journal, 21 April 1973, 144-147.
(3) Barber, D. C.: *Digital Computer Processing of Brain Scans using Principal Components.* Phys. Med. Biol., 1976, Vol. 21, 5, 792-803.
(4) Evans, C. R. *et al: MICKIE — An Automated Interviewing System.* NPL Report Com. 97 December 1977.
(5) Slamecka, V. *et al: MARIS: Knowledge System for Internal Medicine.* Int. Proc. Man., 1977, Vol. 13, 273-276.